MOUSSA ISSA LENDE

BENEFITS OF NUTRITIONAL INTERVENTIONS IN SOUTH KIVU

ScienciaScripts

Imprint

Cover image: www.ingimage.com

This book is a translation from the original published under ISBN 978-620-6-71970-0.

Publisher:
Sciencia Scripts
is a trademark of
Dodo Books Indian Ocean Ltd. and OmniScriptum S.R.L publishing group

120 High Road, East Finchley, London, N2 9ED, United Kingdom
Str. Armeneasca 28/1, office 1, Chisinau MD-2012, Republic of Moldova, Europe
Printed at: see last page
ISBN: 978-620-8-08866-8

MOUSSA ISSA LENDE

BENEFITS OF NUTRITIONAL INTERVENTIONS IN SOUTH KIVU

Table of contents

Preface :

Life, misfortune, isolation, abandonment and poverty are battlefields that have their heroes, obscure heroes sometimes greater than illustrious heroes (Victor Hugo).

According to Thomas Edison, "The doctors of the future will no longer know how to treat the human body with drugs, but rather how to cure and prevent nutrition-related diseases".

In his book, the humanitarian and expert in health and nutrition, Dr Moussa Issa Lende, talks about the benefits of nutritional interventions in South Kivu in the Democratic Republic of Congo in 2020.

In the face of the benefits of humanitarian interventions, it is hard to imagine a greater injustice that deprives children, in the womb and from an early age, of the ability to develop their talents to the full throughout their lives. This represents a violation of their rights, but also an enormous burden for countries whose future citizens will be neither as healthy nor as productive as they could have been (UNICEF, 2013).

However, it is recognised that humanitarian intervention improves the living conditions of vulnerable populations (children, women, the elderly) but this humanitarian assistance does not cover all essential needs. As a result, humanitarian assistance represents only part of what vulnerable populations need to meet their most important needs.

Consequently, the quality of humanitarian assistance and its management by the local authorities are critical factors in beneficiary satisfaction.

This shows that meeting needs does not depend exclusively on donors' humanitarian aid budgets (C. Fabre et al., 2019).

However, if humanitarian assistance is not enough to meet the most important needs of vulnerable populations, it is even less effective in achieving economic self-sufficiency.

However, vulnerable people want to be self-sufficient rather than long-term recipients of humanitarian aid. With this in mind, it is clear that humanitarian assistance in itself should not be used to provoke or end conflicts. However, this same humanitarian assistance can be at the root of conflicts, even inter-community conflicts, which can have the opposite effect to that intended by the humanitarian intervention, if the customs, cultures and traditions of the beneficiaries are not taken into account in these humanitarian interventions.

It is for this reason that humanitarian actors generally find themselves at the heart of important issues requiring humanitarian interventions capable of resolving crisis situations and avoiding humanitarian tragedies. (NGANONGO, 2019).

It is against this backdrop that the author has tackled this issue, which is still a topical subject that has an impact on African development and the healthy survival of young children.

His work is exemplary in more ways than one, and his book is an illustration of the quality of his solid humanitarian experience in several contexts and in several countries (Niger, Mali, Senegal and the Democratic Republic of Congo).

In writing this book about his rich experience in humanitarian aid, the author demonstrates a critical and synthetic spirit in his search for ways to mobilise the resources needed to achieve one of the Sustainable Development Goals: eradicating all forms of malnutrition by empowering beneficiaries while respecting their cultural and traditional values.

Finally, the work of the author from Niger perfectly illustrates that there is high-quality scientific research in Africa carried out by Africans. With this in mind, the author hopes that his book will serve as a stimulus for constructive reflection and a thorough review of the implementation of humanitarian assistance for vulnerable populations in Africa.

Introduction :

Generally speaking, humanitarian assistance is provided as a result of natural disasters, armed conflict, health crises and food crises. The aim of humanitarian assistance is to provide aid to victims of armed conflict and humanitarian crises without discrimination.

As a result, the proliferation of humanitarian crises and disasters is increasing the need for humanitarian aid throughout the world, and particularly in Africa, to meet the need for food, water, medical care and shelter. These humanitarian interventions bring relief to populations suffering from malnutrition, disease, injury, torture, harassment, disappearances, extra-judicial executions and forced displacement.

However, the Democratic Republic of Congo (DRC) remains one of the poorest countries in the world, with 63% of the population living on less than USD 1.25 a day (World Bank, 2018).

In the DRC, undernutrition remains a major public health problem. According to the Food Security and Nutrition Outlook 2022, nearly 2.8 million children under the age of five are likely to suffer from acute malnutrition, and among these children, 887,000 are likely to suffer from severe acute malnutrition. Similarly, 2.2 million pregnant and breastfeeding women are likely to suffer from acute malnutrition in 2022.

In South Kivu, children's diet is characterised by low dietary diversity, inadequate nutritional quality and a low minimum acceptable household diet.

Worse still, in South Kivu, poor dietary practices contribute to a high prevalence of stunted growth in children under 5, and increase their vulnerability to disease through a decline in their immune system.

In South Kivu, according to the nutrition survey (MICS, 2019), the prevalence of underweight is 23% and that of chronic malnutrition is 48%.

In South Kivu, according to the SMART Nutrition Report 2019 and SNSAP (Nutritional Surveillance, Food Security and Early Warning), the territories of Kalehe (Minova), Kabare (Kabare, Bunyakiri, Kalonge), Walungu (Mwana, Mubumbano) and Uvira are facing an alarming nutritional situation. This nutritional situation is exacerbated by food insecurity, inadequate access to quality health services, inappropriate feeding practices for infants, children and women, insufficient diversification of diets and low crop productivity.

In addition, the health zones in the territories of Kalehe (Minova), Kabare (Kabare, Bunyakiri, Kalonge), Walungu (Mwana, Mubumbano) and Uvira are subject to chronic instability linked to clashes between armed groups, which have led to massive population displacements, the destruction of basic socio-economic infrastructure, increased poverty and a sharp deterioration in people's survival mechanisms. In addition, these health zones are often confronted with recurrent epidemics of cholera, measles, Ebola, COVID-19, etc. As a result, social indicators are very low and human rights violations are legion.

The consequences include morbidity and mortality linked to undernutrition, which primarily affects children under five (5) and pregnant and breastfeeding women.

This volatile and alarming situation requires humanitarian nutritional assistance (emergency food distribution) and health care for children (management of cases of global acute malnutrition), which are often accompanied by nutritional promotion activities.

I. Justification for humanitarian assistance (nutrition and healthcare)

In view of this humanitarian situation, the health zones in the territories of Kalehe (Minova), Kabare (Kabare, Bunyakiri, Kalonge), Walungu (Mwana, Mubumbano) and Uvira require both nutritional assistance to reduce the prevention of undernutrition and immediate treatment of child undernutrition. It is essential to improve food security and access to healthcare for vulnerable populations.

However, emergency nutritional action can only make sense if communities and beneficiaries are involved and trained. In this sense, providing the food aid necessary for the survival of the vulnerable can only be effective if it takes account of cultures, traditions, eating habits according to age and the nutritional needs of each individual (reducing chronic deficiencies). For humanitarian assistance to be effective, it is important to build the capacity of health authorities, local authorities and beneficiary communities in order to ensure the recovery (sustainability) of humanitarian interventions.

In order to carry out humanitarian operations successfully, two components are essential: understanding and acceptance by the community and technical expertise.

Humanitarian actors are providing technical support and funding for the implementation of protection programmes, food support, nutritional rehabilitation and food resilience programmes.

Humanitarian actors therefore begin by identifying community leaders and vulnerable groups in the population, but they also work hand in hand with the local authorities, the social partners and the health authorities.

Under this option, a humanitarian intervention focusing on the prevention and treatment of undernutrition, particularly severe acute malnutrition in children under five, is organised for the benefit of children in the form of nutritional and medical assistance on a periodic basis depending on the availability of resources (financial, food, medicines, etc.).

Humanitarian nutritional interventions are generally focused on treating severe acute undernutrition and promoting infant and young child feeding in seventy-four (74) nutritional units in health zones in the territories of Kalehe (Minova), Kabare (Kabare, Bunyakiri, Kalonge), Walungu (Mwana, Mubumbano) and Uvira.

With these humanitarian nutritional interventions, mothers of children take part in activities to promote child health care and in culinary demonstrations, nutritional education and counselling activities with early diagnosis of undernutrition in the villages attached to the health areas.

With the participation of local authorities, health authorities, civil society, humanitarian actors and donors, during the implementation period (one year), the humanitarian nutritional assistance is composed of a prevention component of undernutrition based on the promotion of good nutritional practices and another component of therapeutic care in nutritional units is implemented with a view to saving lives and changing lives.

In order to fully understand the effects and limitations of humanitarian nutritional assistance, the following question is asked: *what is the benefit of humanitarian nutritional interventions in the territories of Kalehe (Minova), Kabare (Kabare, Bunyakiri, Kalonge), Walungu (Mwana, Mubumbano) and Uvira in South Kivu?*

In the same vein, the research has qualified the hypothesis that :

building the capacity of beneficiaries could ensure that the benefits of humanitarian nutritional interventions in South Kivu are sustained over the long term.

To answer this research question and test the research hypothesis, an evaluation of the humanitarian nutrition intervention will be carried out from 19 June 2019 to 20 July 2020 to gather testimonies from beneficiaries on the benefits of the humanitarian nutrition intervention in South Kivu.

The objectives of this study are as follows:

II. Objectives of research into humanitarian nutrition intervention:

2.1- General objective :

Assessing the benefits of the humanitarian nutritional intervention for the vulnerable population of the territories of Kalehe (Minova), Kabare (Kabare, Bunyakiri, Kalonge), Walungu (Mwana, Mubumbano) and Uvira in South Kivu in DR Congo.

2.2- Specific objectives :

- Assess nutritional interventions at health service and community (village) level;
- To determine the practices and knowledge of mothers of children at community level ;
- Evaluating the effects of nutritional practices and child care;
- Documenting good practice and lessons learned to improve the implementation of humanitarian interventions in real time.

III. Methodological approach to the evaluation of humanitarian nutrition interventions :

3.1- Type of survey

This is a descriptive tr yearsversal analytical survey with a comparative aim, whose study population the evaluation of humanitarian intervention is made up of :

- Mother and child pairs aged 0-23 months who took part in cooking demonstration activities
- Mother and child pairs being treated in the UNTA (*Unité Nutritionnelle Thérapeutique Ambulatoire*) and UNTI (*Unité Nutritionnelle Thérapeutique Intensive*) units

3.2- Data collection techniques and tools

The technique used to evaluate the humanitarian intervention is based on a semi-structured interview using an electronic questionnaire for households.

This electronic questionnaire consists of a section collecting information on the identity of mothers of children aged 0 to 23 months and mothers of children treated in UNTA and UNTI in the territories of Kalehe (Minova), Kabare (Kabare, Bunyakiri, Kalonge), Walungu (Mwana, Mubumbano) and Uvira.

The other part of the electronic questionnaire consists of collecting data on the technical aspects of the nutritional intervention.

As a result, the electronic questionnaires are installed on the interviewers' smartphones (tablets) using the ODK Collect application.

In addition, the data collected from the mothers of the children was transmitted online via the interviewers' telephones using ODK Collect software.

Once the data has been collected, it is automatically sent to the server and received in the ODK Collect database. The data is then extracted from the ODK Collect database and processed using Excel before being analysed using SPSS. **3.3- Sampling for the evaluation of the humanitarian response:**

3.3.1- Sample size :

The size of the sample of mothers to be surveyed in 63 health areas. In each health area, ten (10) mother-couples are selected by random draw.

This gave a sample size of around 630 mother-child pairs.

However, during the field survey, the questionnaire was administered to 637 households in 63 clusters, i.e. 10 households per cluster. The number of clusters was determined on the basis of the interviewers' workload and the accessibility of the clusters for one day.

3.3.2- Sampling procedures

Sampling is based on a three-stage cluster survey.

- At the first sampling stage, clusters are selected according to the probability proportional to their size (in this case, the total population of the village). The sampling frames consist of an exhaustive list of villages in each health zone (Mwana, Mubumbano, Kabare and Uvira) grouped by health area with their corresponding populations.
- At the second sampling stage, households are selected by a reasoned choice. The number of households to be surveyed is allocated by village. The choice of the household in the village is random because it is a simple random draw without replacement of the households surveyed among all the households.
- In the third stage of the survey, the mother-child pair to be surveyed is chosen by random draw. If there are several mothers in the plot, one mother is chosen at random (using numbered pieces of paper) to administer the questionnaire.

3.3.3- Organisation of collection :

Composition of the survey teams :

Data for the evaluation of the humanitarian nutrition intervention is collected by interviewers who are recruited to administer questionnaires in households in the health zones. These interviewers are trained in the use of data collection tools and the method of administering questionnaires to beneficiaries for one day before the start of the study. Smartphones/tablets with electronic questionnaires from the ODK Collect (KOBO) application are used to administer questionnaires to beneficiaries in households.

3.3.4- Training of supervisors and interviewers

A one-day training session was organised for sixteen (16) interviewers and four (4) team leaders to familiarise them with the methodology for collecting and administering the questionnaire in households.

3.3.5- Ethical considerations

During the evaluation of the humanitarian nutrition intervention, the objectives and procedures of the survey are explained to community representatives in order to solicit their support and facilitate their participation. At the same time, the moral support of the village dignitaries (village chief, municipal councillors, religious and customary leaders) is obtained.

At the time of the survey, the interviewers and team leaders detailed all the relevant information to the interviewees (heads of households and mothers of children) by way of introduction, with a view to obtaining consent signed by the heads of households and mothers of children before starting to administer the questionnaire. Confidentiality and anonymity are guaranteed during and after the survey. The information collected is transmitted directly to the ODK Collect database, which limits the confidentiality of the information. Thus, the general conditions of use of the ODK Collect tool do not allow data collected in households to be used for personal purposes, let alone shared with third parties.

3.3.6- Organisation of the field survey

The survey took place from 19 June to 20 July 2020 in the territories of Kalehe (Minova), Kabare (Kabare, Bunyakiri, Kalonge), Walungu (Mwana, Mubumbano) and Uvira, with the participation of beneficiary communities, local authorities, health authorities and civil society.

3.3.7- Analysis of collected data

The data collected is entered directly onto smartphones and tablets using the ODK Collect software by the interviewers under the supervision of the team leaders. The data collected is generated directly by the ODK Collect Excel database. The data was thoroughly cleaned, and some variables were corrected. Qualitative and quantitative data are analysed using SPSS version 21.0 software.

3.3.8- Explanation of the calculation of X^2 (Chi-square) in data analysis

The P value is obtained by calculating X^2 (Chi-square).

This X^2 (Chi-square) is a relationship test used to check whether there is a relationship between a risk of exposure and a disease. If its value, the reduced deviation > 1.960, the alpha probability (or significance level p) < 0.05, this means that the link is statistically significant between the disease and the risk of exposure, and there is less than a 5 in 100 chance that the distribution results from chance for a given value of degrees of freedom (ddl).

3.3.9- Data analysis method :

Quantitative and qualitative data are analysed using SPSS version 21 software. Word and Excel are also used to process texts and design tables and graphs.

3.3.10- Limitations of data collection :

The absence of a baseline evaluation makes it difficult to compare the impact of humanitarian nutrition interventions in South Kivu with this evaluation.

IV- Research results

4.1- Socio-demographic characteristics of beneficiaries

Table 1: Socio-demographic characteristics of beneficiaries

Socio-demographic characteristics	Malnourished				P. value
	MAS children (UNTA)		MAS-C children (UNTI)		
Ages of mothers	**(n)**	**(%)**	**(n)**	**(%)**	
[15-19[	24	4	1	5	
[20-29[	315	49	10	53	**0.02**
[30-39[	235	37	7	37	
[40-70[	63	10	1	5	
Marital status	**(n)**	**(%)**	**(n)**	**(%)**	
Single	44	7	2	11	
Monogamous brides	421	66	5	26	
Polygamous brides	81	13	5	26	**<0.001**
Separated/divorced	19	3	4	21	
Common-law union	56	9	1	5	
Widow	16	3	2	11	
Level of education	**(n)**	**(%)**	**(n)**	**(%)**	
No	289	45,4	9	47	
Primary	220	34,5	6	32	0.1
Secondary	127	19,9	4	21	
Higher education	1	**0,2**	0	0	
Mothers' occupations	**(n)**	**(%)**	**(n)**	**(%)**	
Growers	337	**53**	11	58	
Saleswomen	81	13	3	16	
Seamstresses	9	1	1	5	>0.1
Households	194	30	3	16	
Employees	16	3	1	5	
Number of children under 5	**(n)**	**(%)**	**(n)**	**(%)**	
[0-2[	422	66	14	74	0.2
[3-5[	215	34	5	26	

Of the mothers of the children surveyed, 97% were mothers of children in the Unité Nutritionnelle Thérapeutiques Ambulatoire (UNTA), and the average age of these mothers was 25.

The majority of mothers surveyed had an average age of between 20 and 29 years, i.e. 49% of mothers of UNTA children and 53% of mothers of UNTI children. The distribution of mothers of children between age groups was statistically significant between the different ages of mothers of children (p = 0.02).

The majority of women are married monogamously, i.e. 66% of mothers of UNTA children and 26% of mothers of UNTI children. The distribution of marital status between mothers of children is statistically significant (p<0.001).

Mothers who farm are in the majority in UNTI (58%) than in UNTA (53%). The occupation of children's mothers did not differ between the different child health services in UNTA and UNTI (p >0.1).

Most mothers of children in UNTA and UNTI have no level of education and the highest level is 0.2% among mothers of children in UNTA. Nevertheless, the level of education of mothers of children was not statistically significant between the different groups of mothers of children (p = 0.1).

Most of the mothers had children under 2 years of age admitted to care in the two therapeutic nutrition units. However, the number of children did not differ statistically significantly between the different nutritional units (p = 0.2).

The results in Table 1 showed that there was a statistically significant relationship between the marital status of the children's mothers, the ages of the children's mothers and the different malnourished children admitted for care in the different nutritional units (p <0.05). Similarly, the research showed that there was no statistically significant link between level of education, mother's occupation and the number of malnourished children in the different nutritional units (p>0.05).

4.2 Breakdown of patients by nutritional therapy unit

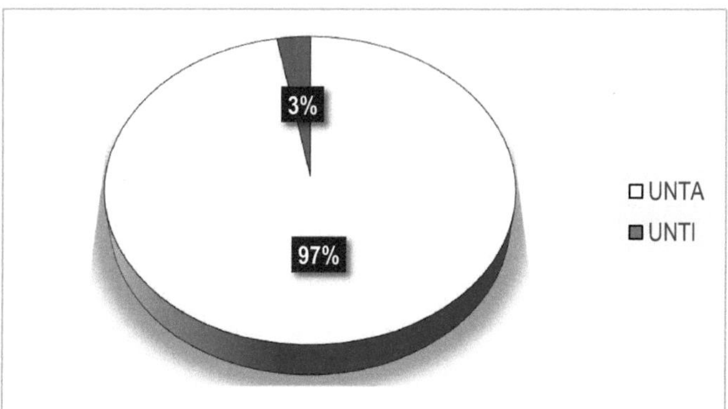

Figure 1: Breakdown of beneficiaries

More mothers of MAS UNTA children (97%) than mothers of MAS-C UNTI children (3%) took part in the study.

4.3 Assessment of nutritional interventions by health and community services

Table 2: Patients by nutritional unit

UNT care	MAS children (UNTA)		MAS-C children (UNTI)		P. value
	(n)	(%)	(n)	(%)	
UNTA	628	99	4	21	**0.0001**
UNTI	9	1	15	79	

99% of MAS children are direct admissions (from screening) to UNTAs, compared with 79% of MAS-C children who are direct admissions to UNITIs.

On the other hand, 21% of MAS children are referred to UNTIs, compared with 1% of MAS-C children who are referred to UNTAs.

The results in table 2 showed that there was a statistically significant relationship between the number of malnourished children and the different nutritional units (UNTA and UNTI) ($p < 0.05$).

Table 3: Assessment of care received by type of malnutrition

Care received	MAS children (UNTA)		MAS-C children (UNTI)		P. value
	(n)	(%)	(n)	(%)	
Excellent	203	32	4	21	0.08
Good	403	63	12	63	
Fair	26	4	3	16	
Mediocre	5	1	0	0	

32% of mothers of MAS children appreciated the care received in the nutritional units more than 21% of mothers of MAS-C children. However, few MAS patients (1%) did not appreciate the care they received, whereas all MAS-C patients appreciated the care they received.

The study showed that there was no statistically significant link between the care provided and the number of malnourished children treated ($p > 0.05$).

Table 4: Assessment of medicines received, by type of malnutrition

Medicines	MAS children (UNTA)		MAS-C children (UNTI)		P. value
	(n)	(%)	(n)	(%)	
Excellent	192	30	7	37	0.8
Good	407	64	11	58	
Fair	26	4	1	5	
Mediocre	12	2	0	0	

37% of mothers of SAM-C children were more appreciative of the medical treatment (receipt of medication) received in the health services compared with 30% of mothers of SAM children. On the other hand, 2% of SAM patients did not appreciate the receipt of medication, whereas all SAM-C patients appreciated the receipt of medication. The study revealed that there was no link between the provision of medicines and the different types of malnourished children treated (p>0.05).

Table 5: Assessment of nutritional inputs received

Nutritional inputs	MAS children (UNTA)		MAS-C children (UNTI)		P. value
	(n)	(%)	(n)	(%)	
Excellent	236	37	10	53	0.5
Good	370	58	8	42	
Fair	26	4	1	5	
Mediocre	5	1	0	0	

53% of mothers of MAS-C children were more appreciative of the nutritional treatment (Plumpy Nut, therapeutic milks) provided during care, compared with 37% of mothers of MAS children.

On the other hand, few mothers of SAM children (1%) did not appreciate the nutritional inputs received, whereas mothers of SAM-C children did appreciate the nutritional inputs received.

There was no statistically significant difference between the assessment of nutritional inputs and the number of malnourished children treated (p>0.05).

Table 6: Assessment of treatment follow-up by type of malnutrition

Treatment follow-up	MAS children (UNTA)		MAS-C children (UNTI)		P. value
	(n)	(%)	(n)	(%)	
Excellent	182	28.6	5	26	0.9
Good	417	65.5	13	68	
Fair	36	5.7	1	5	
Mediocre	2	0.3	0	0	

28.6% of mothers of MAS children appreciated more the follow-up of their children's treatment in the nutritional units, compared with 26% of mothers of MAS-C children. However, 0.3% of SAM children did not appreciate the follow-up in the nutritional units. The results in Table 6 showed that there was no statistically significant relationship between treatment follow-up and the number of malnourished children ($p>0.05$).

Table 7: Assessment of reception in care departments according to type of malnutrition

Reception at UNT	MAS children (UNTA)		MAS-C children (UNTI)		P. value
	(n)	(%)	(n)	(%)	
Excellent	177	27.8	5	26	0.6
Good	416	65.3	14	74	
Fair	42	6.6	0	0	
Mediocre	2	0.3	0	0	

27.8% of mothers of MAS children in the UNTA appreciated the welcome they received in the health services, compared with 26% of mothers of MAS-C patients in the UNTI. The study showed that there was no statistically significant link between the reception of mothers and the number of malnourished children ($p>0.05$).

Table 8: Assessment of counselling received by type of malnutrition

Counselings	MAS children (UNTA)		MAS-C children (UNTI)		P. value
	(n)	(%)	(n)	(%)	
Excellent	173	27	4	21	0.9
Good	431	68	14	74	
Fair	29	5	1	5	
Mediocre	4	1	0	0	

27% of mothers of SAM children appreciated the counselling received in the health services more than 21% of mothers of SAM-C patients. On the other hand, few mothers of SAM children (1%) appreciated the counselling less.

The study revealed that there was no statistically significant link between the counselling received and the different types of malnourished children (p>0.05).

4.4 Determining the practices and knowledge of mothers at community level

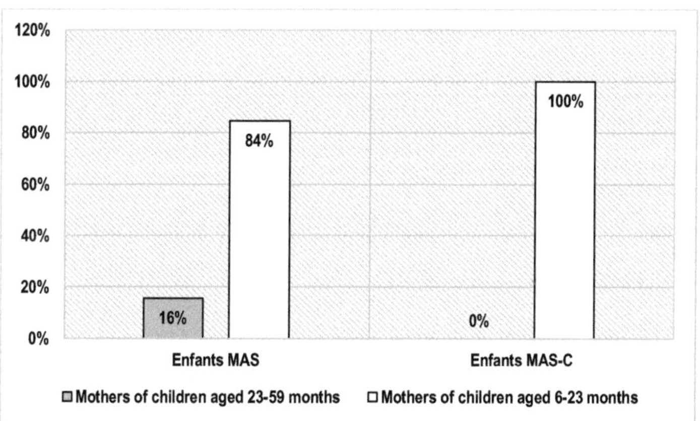

Figure 2: Distribution of malnourished children by unit

All children under two treated in the NICUs are severely acutely malnourished with medical complications. On the other hand, the majority of children treated in the UNTA are severely malnourished without complications under the age of two.

Consequently, there was no statistical relationship between the age distribution of malnourished children and the different therapeutic nutritional units for treating children (p = 0.4).

Table 9: Participation in community activities

Community nutrition	Mothers of children 0-23 months		Mothers of children 23-59 months		P. value
Screenings	**(n)**	**(%)**	**(n)**	**(%)**	
Participants	478	86	85	84	0.6
Non-participants	77	14	16	16	
Cooking demonstration	**(n)**	**(%)**	**(n)**	**(%)**	
Participants	389	81	72	85	0.6
Non-participants	89	19	13	15	
ANJE	**(n)**	**(%)**	**(n)**	**(%)**	
Participants	257	54	47	55	0.8
Non-participants	221	46	38	45	
Nutritional education	**(n)**	**(%)**	**(n)**	**(%)**	
Participants	400	84	74	87	0.6
Non-participants	78	16	11	13	

86% of mothers of children aged 0-23 months were more involved in screening, compared with 84% of mothers of children aged 23-59 months.

85% of mothers of children aged 23-59 months participated more in cooking demonstration activities, compared with 81% of mothers of children aged 0-23 months.

Mothers of children (55%) aged 23-59 months participated more in ANJE promotion activities than mothers of children (54%) aged 0-23 months.

Mothers of children over 23 months old (87%) were more likely to take part in nutrition education activities than mothers of children under two years old (84%).

The above table showed that there was no statistically significant relationship between participation in community nutrition activities (screening sessions, cooking demonstration sessions, ANJE practice sessions) and the different mother-child groups (p>0.05).

Table 10: Assessment of beneficiaries' nutritional education programmes

Appreciation of nutritional education	Children 0-23 months		Children aged 24-59 months		P. value
	(n)	(%)	(n)	(%)	
Excellent	180	38	29	34	
Good	285	60	54	64	0.8
Fair	10	2	2	2	
Mediocre	3	1	0	0	

Mothers of children aged 0-23 months (38%) appreciated nutrition education more than mothers of children aged 24-59 months (34%).

In addition, the study established that there was no statistically significant link between assessments of nutritional education and the different groups of mothers of children ($p>0.05$).

Table 11: Appreciation of cooking demonstrations

Appreciation of culinary demonstrations	Children 0-23 months		Children aged 24-59 months		P. value
	(n)	(%)	(n)	(%)	
Excellent	137	29	29	34	
Good	273	57	52	61	0.1
Fair	27	6	2	2	
Mediocre	41	9	2	2	

34% of mothers of children aged 24-59 months enjoyed the cooking demonstrations more, compared with 29% of mothers of children aged 0-23 months. While 9% of mothers of children aged 0-23 months enjoyed the cooking demonstrations less.

The study showed that there was no statistically significant difference between the assessments of the cooking demonstrations and the different groups of mothers of children ($p>0.05$).

Table 12: Assessment of counselling sessions

Assessment of counselling	Children 0-23 months		Children aged 24-59 months		P. value
	(n)	(%)	(n)	(%)	
Excellent	109	23	21	25	0.3
Good	279	58	53	62	
Fair	40	8	8	9	
Mediocre	50	10	3	4	

25% of mothers of children aged 24-59 months appreciated the counselling more, compared with 23% of mothers of children aged 0-23 months. On the other hand, 10% of mothers of children aged 0-23 months were less appreciative of the counselling they received in the health facilities.

The table above showed that there was no statistical link between the assessments of the counselling received and the assessments of the various mothers of the children ($p>0.05$).

4.5 Assessing the effects of nutritional practices and childcare

Table 13: Practices and knowledge of mothers with children

Practice and knowledge	Mothers of children 0-23 months		Mothers of children 24-59 months		P. value
Causes and consequences of undernutrition	**(n)**	**(%)**	**(n)**	**(%)**	
Included	295	62	55	65	0.7
Not included	183	38	30	35	
Preventing care practices	**(n)**	**(%)**	**(n)**	**(%)**	
Discoveries	281	59	53	62	0.7
Undiscovered	197	41	32	38	
Nutritional value of local products	**(n)**	**(%)**	**(n)**	**(%)**	
Discoveries	299	63	47	55	0.3
Undiscovered	179	37	38	45	
Composition of nutritional meals	**(n)**	**(%)**	**(n)**	**(%)**	
Discoveries	340	71	64	75	0.6
Undiscovered	138	29	21	25	
Nutritious local food recipes	**(n)**	**(%)**	**(n)**	**(%)**	
Discoveries	305	64	56	66	0.8
Undiscovered	173	36	29	34	
Optimum breastfeeding	**(n)**	**(%)**	**(n)**	**(%)**	
Practised	238	50	25	29	0.002
Not practised	240	50	60	71	
Community activities	**(n)**	**(%)**	**(n)**	**(%)**	
Participating	463	97	84	99	0.5
Not participating	15	3	1	1	
Breastfeeding practice	**(n)**	**(%)**	**(n)**	**(%)**	
Mastered	292	61	34	40	0.001
Not mastered	186	39	51	60	

65% of mothers of children aged 24-59 months understood more about the causes and consequences of undernutrition, compared with 62% of mothers of children aged 0-23 months. The understanding of the causes and consequences of undernutrition between the different mothers of children was not statistically significant (p = 0.7).

62% of mothers of children aged 24-59 months discovered more optimal care practices aimed at preventing undernutrition than mothers of children aged 0-23 months (59%). The discovery of optimal care practices between different mothers of children was not statistically significant (p = 0.7).

The nutritional value of local foods was discovered by 63% of mothers of children aged 0-23 months compared with 55% of mothers of children aged 24-59 months. The discovery of the nutritional value of local foods by different mothers of children was not statistically significant (p = 0.6).

The composition of nutritional meals was discovered more by 75% of mothers of children aged 24-59 months than by 71% of mothers of children aged 0-23 months. The discovery of the composition of nutritional meals between the different mothers of children was not statistically significant (p = 0.3).

66% of mothers of children aged 24-59 months discovered more nutritious recipes, compared with 64% of mothers of children aged 0-23 months. There was no statistical significance (p = 0.8) in the discovery of nutritious recipes between the different mothers of children.

Optimal breastfeeding was practised more by mothers of children aged 0-23 months (50%) than by mothers of children aged 24-59 months (29%). Optimal breastfeeding was statistically significant (p = 0.002) among mothers of different babies.

Mothers of children aged 24-59 months (99%) participated more in community nutrition activities than mothers of children aged 0-23 months (97%). Participation in community nutrition activities by mothers of different children was not statistically significant (p = 0.5).

Breastfeeding was better practised by 61% of mothers of children aged 0-23 months compared with 40% of mothers of children aged 24-59 months. Mastery of breastfeeding among the different mothers of children was statistically significant ($p = 0.001$).

However, the study revealed that there was no statistically significant relationship between understanding the causes and consequences of undernutrition, optimal care practice, the nutritional value of foods, the composition of nutritional meals, nutritious recipes, participation in nutrition activities and the different mothers of children ($p>0.05$).

Nevertheless, the study established that there was a statistically significant link between mastery of breastfeeding practice, optimal AM practice and different mothers of children ($p <0.05$).

Table 14: Improving care and nutritional practices

Improving practices	Children 0-23 months		Children 24-59 months		P. value
Weight measurement	**(n)**	**(%)**	**(n)**	**(%)**	
Recorded catch	416	90	76	90	0.9
Unrecorded catch	47	10	8	10	
Disease frequency	**(n)**	**(%)**	**(n)**	**(%)**	
Less sick	286	62	51	61	0.9
Often ill	177	38	33	39	
Crying frequency	**(n)**	**(%)**	**(n)**	**(%)**	
Less	233	50	40	48	0.8
Often	230	50	44	52	
Feeding assessment	**(n)**	**(%)**	**(n)**	**(%)**	
Appetite	346	75	63	75	0.9
No appetite	117	25	21	25	
Smooth latch	**(n)**	**(%)**	**(n)**	**(%)**	
Improved	202	44	13	15	0.0001
Improved to do	261	56	71	85	

Weight gain was proportionally (90%) equal between the group of mothers with children and this weight gain was not statistically significant between the two groups of mothers with children ($p = 0.9$).

Appetite was proportionally better (75%) between the group of mothers with children and this weight gain was not statistically significant between the two groups of mothers with children ($p = 0.9$).

Children aged 0-23 months (62%) are less likely to fall ill than children aged 24-59 months (61%).

Children aged 0-23 months cry less (50%) than children aged 24-59 months (48%).

Children aged 0-23 months (44%) took to the breast better without difficulty than children aged 24-59 months (15%).

However, there was no statistically significant relationship between weight measurement, frequency of illness, diet assessment and the different ages of the children ($p>0.05$).

However, there was a statistically significant link between nutritional practices and the different ages of the children ($p < 0.05$).

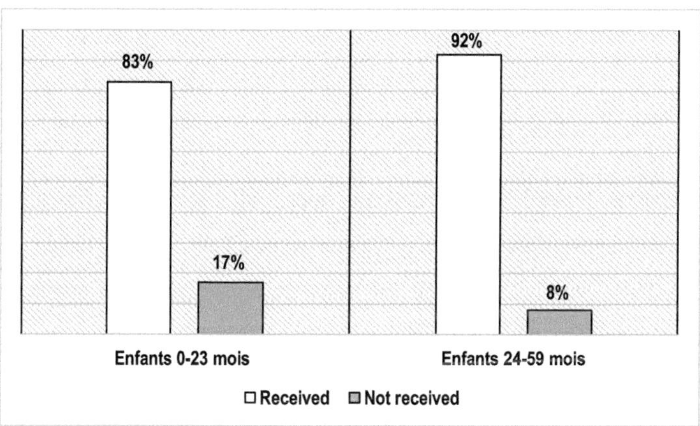

Figure 3: Home visits for cooking demonstrations

Mothers of children aged 24-59 months (92%) received more home visits to assess their cooking demonstration practices than mothers of children aged 0-23 months (83%).

On the other hand, 17% of children aged 0-23 months were visited more frequently for follow-up of nutritional treatment at home.

Table 15: Assessment of home visits

Appreciation of home visits	Children 0-23 months		Children aged 24-59 months		P. value
	(n)	(%)	(n)	(%)	
Excellent	110	28	15	19	0.3
Good	274	69	60	77	
Fair	3	1	2	3	
Mediocre	9	2	1	1	

Mothers of children aged 0-23 months (28%) appreciated the home visits more for their cooking demonstrations than mothers of children aged 24-59 months (19%).

Furthermore, there was no statistical link between community food practices and the different ages of children ($p>0.05$).

Table 16: Capacity building for health and nutrition care

Capacity building	Mothers of children 0-23 months		Mothers of children 24-59 months		P. value
Care and nutrition practices	**(n)**	**(%)**	**(n)**	**(%)**	
Received	396	83	78	92	0.7
Not received	82	17	7	8	

Mothers of children aged 24-59 months (92%) received more capacity building on health care, hygiene and nutritional practices than mothers of children aged 0-23 months (83%). The results of this table showed that there was no link between capacity building and the different ages of the children ($p>0.05$).

Table 17: Assessment of capacity building

Appreciation of capacity building	Children 0-23 months		Children aged 24-59 months		P. value
	(n)	(%)	(n)	(%)	
Excellent	110	26	12	16	0.2
Good	301	72	61	80	
Fair	7	2	3	4	
Mediocre	1	0	0	0	

26% of mothers of children aged 0-23 months appreciated the capacity building they received at home, compared with 16% of mothers of children aged 24-59 months.

According to the results of the study, there was no statistically significant difference between the capacity-building practices and the different mother-child groups ($p>0.05$).

V. Discussion of the results :

5.1 Assessment of nutritional interventions in health services

In terms of appreciation of the nutritional interventions, mothers of SAM children admitted to the UNTA were more appreciative of the care received in the therapeutic nutritional units (health services) than were mothers of MAS-C children in the UNTI.

Secondly, the mothers of MAS patients at the UNTA were more appreciative of the treatment follow-up for the children they cared for, compared with the mothers of MAS-C children at the UNTI.

In addition, the mothers of MAS patients from the UNTA were more appreciative of the welcome they received in the health services than the mothers of MAS-C children from the UNTI.

Finally, the mothers of MAS children at the UNTA were more appreciative of the counselling they received during care than the mothers of MAS-C children at the UNTI.

On the other hand, mothers of SAM-C children admitted to the UNTI were more appreciative of the medical treatment (receipt of medication) received in the health services than were mothers of SAM children in the UNTA.

In addition, the mothers of MAS-C children in the UNTI were more appreciative of the nutritional treatment (Plumpy Nut, therapeutic milks) they received during care than the mothers of MAS children in the UNTA.

According to the statistical analysis, there is no significant statistical relationship ($p>0.05$) between the care received, the follow-up of children's treatment, the reception in the health services, the counselling received during care, the medical treatment (receipt of medication) received, the nutritional treatment (receipt of Plumpy Nut, therapeutic milks) received and the different groups of malnourished children treated in the UNTAs and in the UNTIs.

5.2 Practices and knowledge of mothers at community and household level

In terms of knowledge, mothers of children aged 24-59 months were more aware of the causes and consequences of undernutrition than mothers of children aged 0-23 months.

In practical terms, mothers of children aged 24-59 months practised more optimal care aimed at preventing undernutrition than mothers of children aged 0-23 months.

In terms of feeding children and pregnant women, mothers of children aged between 24 and 59 months discovered more nutritional meals prepared during cooking demonstrations in communities and households.

As a result, mothers of children aged 0-23 months discovered more about the nutritional value of local foods than mothers of children aged 24-59 months.

In terms of breastfeeding, mothers of children aged 0-23 months were more likely to practise optimal breastfeeding (breastfeeding within half an hour of birth, exclusive breastfeeding and continuous breastfeeding) than mothers of children aged 24-59 months.

Mothers of children aged 0-23 months mastered good breastfeeding practices better than mothers of children aged 24-59 months.

Optimal breastfeeding practice and mastery of breastfeeding practice were statistically related to the practices and knowledge of mothers of children at community and household level ($p < 0.05$). On the other hand, understanding the causes and consequences of undernutrition, optimal care practices, the nutritional value of foods, the composition of nutritional meals, nutritious recipes and participation in community nutrition activities were statistically unrelated to the practices and knowledge of mothers at community and household level ($p > 0.05$).

5.3 Improving nutritional practices and childcare by mothers of children

In terms of care, children aged 0-23 months fell less ill than children aged 24-59 months. Secondly, in terms of indicators of children's well-being, children aged 0-23 months cried less than children aged 24-59 months.

In terms of promoting breastfeeding, children aged 0-23 months were more likely to latch on without difficulty than children aged 24-59 months.

Finally, in terms of nutrition, mothers of children aged 24-59 months received more home visits to assess cooking demonstration practices with a view to improving the nutrition of children in the home. On the other hand, children aged 0-23 months received the most home visits to improve the monitoring of nutritional treatment at home. As a result, mothers of children aged 0-23 months appreciated the home visits more to assess their take-up of cooking demonstrations at home than mothers of children aged 24-59 months.

However, weight measurement, frequency of illness and diet assessment were not statistically related to improvements in nutritional practices and child care provided by the groups of mothers with children ($p>0.05$).

While breastfeeding without difficulty was statistically linked to improved nutritional practices and childcare by mothers ($p <0.05$).

5.4 Capacity-building for mothers to ensure the sustainability of achievements

In terms of capacity building, mothers of children aged 24-59 months received more capacity building than mothers of children aged 0-23 months.

Mothers of children aged between 24 and 59 months received more capacity-building on good health care practices for children, but they also received capacity-building on good hygiene practices, good feeding practices, good breastfeeding promotion practices and nutritional practices.

On the other hand, mothers of children aged 0-23 months who received less capacity building were the ones who appreciated the capacity building received at home more than mothers of children aged 24-59 months.

Lastly, there was no statistical link between capacity building and sustainability ($p>0.05$).

Conclusion:

At the end of the research, it should be noted that the benefits of nutritional interventions for the population of South Kivu in the Democratic Republic of Congo made it possible firstly to assess nutritional interventions at health service and community level, then to determine the practices and knowledge of mothers of children at community level, then to assess the effects of nutritional practices and child care by mothers of children and finally to document good practices and lessons learned to improve the implementation of humanitarian interventions.

Next, the benefit of nutritional interventions revealed that breastfeeding was better practised by mothers of children aged 0-23 months than by mothers of children aged 24-59 months. The benefit of the nutritional interventions showed that optimal breastfeeding was practised more by mothers of children aged 0-23 months than by mothers of children aged 24-59 months.

In addition, the benefits of the nutritional interventions showed that children aged 0-23 months latched on better without difficulty than children aged 24-59 months.

However, mothers of children aged 24-59 months received more capacity-building on good nutritional practices, health care and good feeding practices than mothers of children aged 0-23 months.

Finally, optimal breastfeeding practice, mastery of breastfeeding practice and taking the breast without difficulty have a statistical relationship with the capacity building received by the different mothers of children ($p < 0.05$). On the other hand, the appreciation of nutritional interventions at the level of health services and the capacity building of mothers to ensure the sustainability of what they have learned have no statistical link with the practices and knowledge of mothers at the community and household levels ($p > 0.05$).

Practical suggestions :

With regard to the issue of sustaining the achievements of nutritional interventions, it would be essential to give responsibility for managing nutritional interventions to the beneficiaries (mothers of children). This transfer of responsibility to mothers must be accompanied by the regeneration of income to promote access to healthcare, access to food and the fight against infectious diseases in children under the supervision of local (health) authorities with the participation of humanitarian actors. It is also essential to focus on the continued promotion of breastfeeding and infant and child feeding, whatever the type of humanitarian intervention and whatever the humanitarian context (conflict, humanitarian crisis, development, etc.). It would also be important to improve the nutrition of mothers and children, while improving hygiene and sanitation (parasite control) through household water treatment, the promotion of handwashing with soap at home, the use of mosquito nets and periodic deworming of children. It would also be essential to promote the consumption of micronutrient-rich foods by preparing food for children in the community. It would also be important to focus on the treatment of sick children in health services.

Lastly, it would be very beneficial to guarantee the availability and diversification of food. To achieve this, it is vital to strengthen agricultural production through local production of food at home, transfers and safety nets, and the strengthening of local purchasing from small farmers. But we also need to monitor the issue of overweight mothers and children in the event of overnutrition in humanitarian interventions.

Declaration of competing interests

The author declares that he has no known competing financial interests or personal relationships that might appear to influence the work presented in this book.

Data availability :

For reasons of deontology and ethical considerations, the information collected is treated anonymously and confidentially and its sharing is not authorised.

Acknowledgements :

To the interviewers, health authorities and local authorities who facilitated data collection in the health areas and in the communities (households).

The respondents (mothers of children) who took part in the research and provided answers during data collection in their households.

To all those who gave their encouragement and unfailing support for the writing of the book.

References :

C. Fabre et al (2019). Living in crisis: what do beneficiaries of humanitarian aid tell us? https://defishumanitaires.com/2019/10/17/vivre-en-situation-de-crise-que-nous-disent-les-beneficiaires-.

NGANONGO, O. (2019). Development projects in sub-Saharan Africa, between social change and social norms,. *Revue Africaine de Sociologie, Vol. 23, No. 2 (2019), pp. 147-159 (13 pages), Published By: CODESRIA,* https://www.jstor.org/stable/2686808, pp. 147-159 (13 pages).

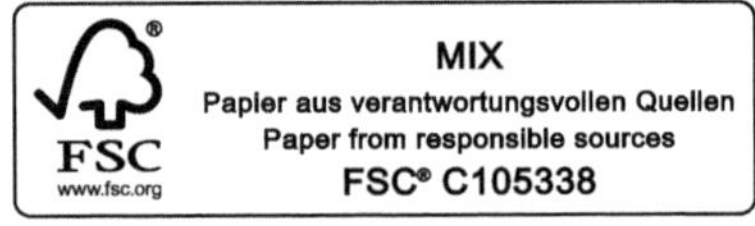

Printed by Books on Demand GmbH, Norderstedt / Germany